Enlarged Prostate?

Treatment.

Table of contents

Introduction

Step into a world where the whispers of vulnerability meet the triumph of modern medical science. In the pages of "Enlarged Prostate? Treatment," embark on a captivating journey that unveils the secrets to reclaiming control over your health and restoring the symphony of life's precious moments.

Within the confines of this remarkable book, a symphony conductor of knowledge and compassion, you will find yourself immersed in an enchanting narrative that transcends the boundaries of a simple medical guide. It is a tale of hope, resilience, and the indomitable human spirit, woven with the threads of expertise and understanding.

Prepare to be captivated as you uncover a wealth of invaluable information, illuminating the path to conquering the challenges posed by an enlarged prostate. Whether you are the afflicted individual seeking solace, a caring companion lending support, or a curious soul yearning for knowledge, this literary masterpiece is a beacon of enlightenment.

Through meticulous research and the insights of leading experts in the field, this book serves as your guiding star, illuminating the maze of treatment options and empowering you to make informed decisions. It goes beyond the surface, delving into the intricacies of the condition, unraveling the myths, and unveiling the latest breakthroughs that promise respite from the clutches of discomfort.

Yet, "Enlarged Prostate? Treatment" is not merely a compendium of facts and figures. It possesses a magical quality, gently guiding you through stories of real-life heroes who have stood tall in the face of adversity. Their triumphs will inspire you to embrace the notion that every setback can be transformed into an opportunity for growth, and every challenge surmountable with the right knowledge and determination.

As you turn each page, the book becomes your trusted confidant, sympathetically addressing your concerns and offering a comforting hand to steady your path. With clarity and compassion, it provides a roadmap towards a brighter tomorrow, where the symphony of your life reverberates harmoniously once more.

So, fellow seekers of knowledge, prepare to embark on a transformational voyage through the pages of "Enlarged Prostate? Treatment." Let its enchanting prose and expert guidance dance upon your senses, as you discover the power within you to embrace a life free from the shackles of an enlarged prostate.

Helpful Quotes and Advice on Prostate Enlargement

"Treatment for prostate enlargement depends on the severity of symptoms and individual circumstances. Options range from lifestyle changes to medication or surgical intervention."

"Alpha-blockers, such as tamsulosin or terazosin, are commonly prescribed medications that can help relax the muscles in the prostate and bladder neck, improving urine flow."

"5-alpha reductase inhibitors, like finasteride or dutasteride, may be used to shrink the prostate gland by reducing the production of hormones that contribute to its enlargement."

"Minimally invasive procedures, such as transurethral microwave therapy (TUMT) or prostate artery embolization (PAE), are alternative options for treating prostate enlargement and can offer relief from symptoms."

"In severe cases or when other treatments have not been effective, surgical procedures like transurethral resection of the prostate (TURP) or laser ablation may be recommended to remove or reduce the size of the prostate."

"Lifestyle modifications, such as limiting fluid intake before bedtime, avoiding caffeine and alcohol, and practicing pelvic floor exercises, can help manage symptoms associated with prostate enlargement."

Remember, these quotes are not exhaustive and should not replace professional medical advice. Consulting a healthcare provider will provide you with the most accurate and suitable treatment options for your specific situation.

Chapter One

Causes Of Prostate Enlargement

It is important to understand the possible causes of prostate enlargement, in order to know what to do to overcome the problem.

First and foremost, what is prostate enlargement?

Prostate enlargement, also known as benign prostatic hyperplasia (BPH), is a common condition that affects many men as they age. Infact it is the most common prostate problem in males over 50. This is simply when the Prostate Gland has grown too large that its size presses and pinches the urethra, narrowing the urethra tube. This makes it difficult for urine to pass and mostly leads to other problems.

While the exact cause of BPH is not fully understood, several factors may contribute to its development. Mentioned below are some possible causes.

- Hormonal changes: As men age, their hormone levels change, particularly their levels of testosterone and estrogen. These hormonal changes can cause the prostate gland to grow larger.

- Age: BPH is more common in older men. As men age, their prostate gland grows in size, which can put pressure on the urethra and lead to symptoms of BPH.

- Family history: Men with a family history of BPH may be more likely to develop the condition themselves.

- Lifestyle factors: Certain lifestyle factors, such as a diet high in saturated fats, lack of exercise, and obesity, may increase the risk of developing BPH.

- Other medical conditions: Certain medical conditions, such as diabetes, heart disease, and high blood pressure, may increase the risk of developing BPH.

It is important to note that while prostate enlargement is common, it can also be a symptom of prostate cancer. If you experience any symptoms of BPH, such as difficulty urinating or a weak urine stream, it is important to see a doctor to rule out any underlying medical conditions.

Prevention: Prostate Enlargement

Prostate enlargement, also known as benign prostatic hyperplasia (BPH), is a common condition in men, particularly in older men. While there is no guaranteed way to prevent BPH from occurring, there are several lifestyle changes and medical interventions that can help reduce the risk of developing the condition or reduce its severity.

- Maintain a healthy weight: Being overweight or obese can increase the risk of developing BPH. Therefore, maintaining a healthy weight through regular exercise and a balanced diet can help reduce the risk of BPH.

- Exercise regularly: Regular exercise has been shown to reduce the risk of BPH. Exercise helps to maintain a healthy weight and improves overall health and wellbeing.

- Eat a healthy diet: Eating a diet that is rich in fruits, vegetables, and whole grains has been associated with a reduced risk of BPH. Conversely, diets that are high in red meat and fat may increase the risk of BPH.

- Limit alcohol consumption: Drinking alcohol excessively can increase the risk of BPH. Men should limit their alcohol consumption to no more than two drinks per day.

- Quit smoking: Smoking has been linked to an increased risk of BPH. Therefore, quitting smoking can help reduce the risk of developing the condition.

- Reduce stress: Stress can contribute to a range of health problems, including BPH. Finding ways to reduce stress, such as through meditation, yoga, or other relaxation techniques, can help reduce the risk of BPH.

- Regularly screen for prostate cancer: Men over the age of 50 should get screened for prostate cancer regularly. While prostate cancer and BPH are not directly related, the symptoms of both conditions are similar. Therefore, getting regular screenings can help identify any potential problems early on.

In summary, while there is no guaranteed way to prevent BPH, maintaining a healthy weight, exercising regularly, eating a healthy diet, limiting alcohol consumption, quitting smoking, reducing stress, regularly screening for prostate cancer, taking medication, and considering surgery can all help reduce the risk of developing BPH or reduce the severity of symptoms. It is important to discuss any concerns about BPH with a doctor to determine the best course of action.

Urine Retention & Prostate Enlargement

Urine retention in the bladder can contribute to prostate enlargement through a variety of mechanisms. The prostate gland surrounds the urethra, which is the tube that carries urine from the bladder out of the body. When the prostate gland becomes enlarged, it can put pressure on the urethra and interfere with the normal flow of urine. This can lead to incomplete emptying of the bladder and urine retention.

Chronic urine retention can lead to increased pressure and tension within the bladder, which can cause it to become distended and enlarged over time. This can also lead to stretching and weakening of the bladder muscles, which can further contribute to urine retention and exacerbate prostate enlargement.

In addition, urine retention can increase the risk of urinary tract infections (UTIs), which can also contribute to prostate enlargement. UTIs can cause inflammation and damage to the prostate gland, leading to swelling and enlargement.

Conclusively, urine retention in the bladder can contribute to prostate enlargement through a complex interplay of mechanical, muscular, and inflammatory factors. It is important to seek medical attention if you experience symptoms of prostate enlargement or urinary retention, as prompt diagnosis and treatment can help prevent complications and improve outcomes.

Chapter Two

Treatment Of Prostate Enlargement

Prostate enlargement, also known as benign prostatic hyperplasia (BPH), is a common condition that can cause urinary symptoms such as frequent urination, urgency, weak stream, and difficulty starting or stopping urine flow. Treatment for prostate enlargement depends on the severity of symptoms, the size of the prostate, and the patient's overall health.

Stated below are some common treatment options for prostate enlargement.

- Watchful waiting: If the symptoms are mild or moderate, a doctor may recommend watchful waiting, which means monitoring the condition and waiting to see if the symptoms worsen.

- Medications: Several medications can help relieve the symptoms of prostate enlargement. These include alpha-blockers, which relax the muscles in the prostate and bladder neck to improve urine flow, and 5-alpha reductase inhibitors, which reduce the size of the prostate gland. Other medications that can be used include anticholinergics, phosphodiesterase-5 inhibitors, and combination therapies.

- Minimally invasive procedures: There are several minimally invasive procedures that can be used to treat prostate enlargement, such as transurethral resection of the prostate (TURP), laser therapy, and microwave therapy. These procedures involve removing or shrinking the prostate tissue to improve urine flow.

A true life experience on how Minimally invasive procedures were used to treat prostate enlargement.

Paul is a healthy, average-looking 57-year-old. He is active in his neighborhood and volunteers at his son's high school. He also appreciates outdoor sports and excursions. Paul has had prostate troubles in recent years, notably an enlarged prostate, also known as benign prostatic hyperplasia (BPH), which has limited his ability to fully enjoy the things he enjoys.

"When you have BPH, your life revolves around your bladder and the nearest bathroom," Paul says. "You get tired of standing for long periods of time waiting to use the restroom, you wake up several times a night, and you have to adjust your liquid intake because you won't be near a bathroom for a few hours."

Paul's health deteriorated when he was on holiday with his family. Paul and his kid were on a camping trip whitewater rafting when he began to experience significant discomfort when he needed to use the lavatory. He recalls needing to use the restroom all the time, but once they stopped for a break, he could barely urinate. After a day of this, his symptoms worsened to the point where he couldn't urinate even when he was in great pain. Paul was taken to a nearby hospital after another agonizing 24 hours.

"Things like breathing, eating, sleeping, and waste disposal are things we take for granted," Paul explains. "You don't really understand what it's like until you've been on the other side."

The doctor Paul met while abroad placed a catheter as a temporary remedy until he could return home to treat his pressing issue. When he arrived home, he immediately saw his doctor. Paul's doctor referred him to Dr. Frank Lai after he had been living with a catheter for two months.

"Dr. Lai was recommended to me by my doctor as being fantastic and insanely smart. "He said Dr. Lai was the person to see for urology," Paul recalls. Following their initial consultation, Dr. Lai advised him for AquaBeam Waterjet Ablation Therapy. Paul was quickly scheduled for the minimally invasive treatment at El Camino Health's Los Gatos hospital.

Aquablation treatment is a surgical procedure used to treat lower urinary tract infections.

Paul stayed in the hospital for one night following the procedure. "I will never forget my interactions with the doctors and nurses who assisted me." Following my operation, I was completely reliant on them, and they were fantastic. "I could tell they didn't just do it because it was their job, but because they cared about me and how I was doing," Paul adds.

He was discharged with a urinary catheter, which was removed at a follow-up consultation. Paul was able to resume his normal activities within a few days and after consulting with Dr. Lai. Paul has now been out of the hospital for nine months and feels like he has reclaimed his life.

Aquablation completely changes the game. While it isn't life or death, it has "certainly been the difference between a life that isn't worth living and a life that you're very happy to be living," Paul says. "I would advise anyone suffering from BPH to not wait. I am eternally grateful to Dr. Lai and the El Camino staff. They restored my life."

- Surgery: In some cases, surgery may be necessary to treat prostate enlargement. The most common surgical procedure is a prostatectomy, which involves removing part or all of the prostate gland, which can help relieve symptoms. However, surgery carries risks, so it is important to discuss the potential benefits and risks of surgery with a doctor before undergoing the procedure.

It's important to discuss the risks and benefits of each treatment option with your doctor to determine the best course of action for your individual situation.

Herbs and plants that can be used to treat prostate enlargement

Prostate enlargement, also known as benign prostatic hyperplasia (BPH), is a common condition that affects many men as they age. While there are many conventional medical treatments available for BPH, some men may be interested in exploring natural remedies, including herbs and plants. Here are some herbs and plants that have been traditionally used to treat prostate enlargement.

- Saw Palmetto: Saw palmetto is one of the most popular natural remedies for BPH. It is essential to prostate healing and works by reducing the conversion of testosterone to dihydrotestosterone (DHT), which is responsible for prostate growth. Saw palmetto has been shown to reduce symptoms such as frequent urination, weak urine flow, and incomplete bladder emptying.

- Pygeum: Pygeum is a tree native to Africa whose bark has been used for centuries to treat urinary problems. It has been found to reduce inflammation in the prostate gland and improve the urinary system in men.

- Stinging Nettle: Stinging nettle is a plant that has been used for centuries to treat urinary problems. It has been found to reduce inflammation in the prostate gland and improve urinary symptoms in men with BPH.

- Rye Grass Pollen Extract: Rye grass pollen extract has been shown to reduce the size of the prostate gland

and improve urinary symptoms in men with BPH.

- Pumpkin Seed: Pumpkin seeds have been used for centuries to promote prostate health. They are rich in zinc, which is essential for prostate function, and have been shown to relieve urinary symptoms in males suffering from BPH.

- Scorpion tail plant: This plant is essential in the treatment of prostate enlargement.

The picture is shown below:

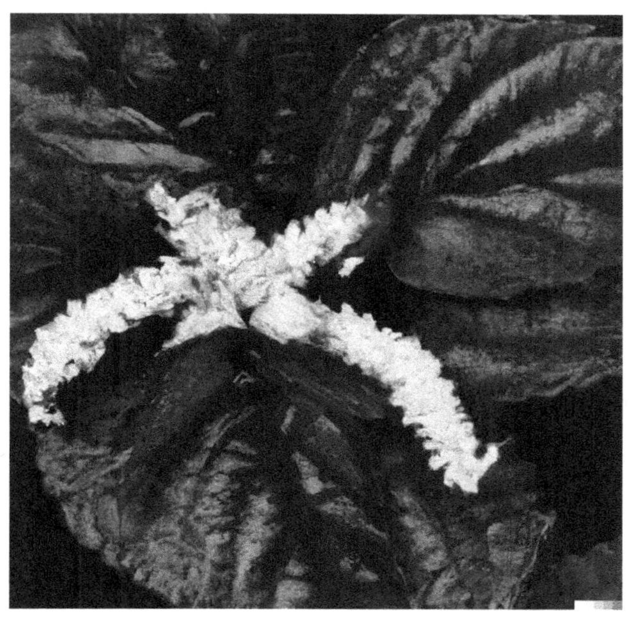

You can take a little quantity (about 20 ml to 40ml) of the juice extracted from it, morning and evening at least for three days. To make it better l recommend to take this extracted juice with a lot of water.

- Turmeric and Garlic : These two herbs are very important for our general health and well being. They can be eaten raw or can be combined with your meal at the point of eating.

I recommend you make them a routine part of your meal on a daily basis by adding them to your food preferably in dry and powdered form. It will certainly help to fight prostate enlargement.

It's important to note that while these herbs and plants may be effective for most men, they are not a substitute for medical treatment, if you are experiencing symptoms of enlarged prostate.

9 798396 415508